MW00917018

The Dr. Scotti Diet

A GUIDE TO LIFELONG WEIGHT CONTROL

Angelo T Scotti, M.D.

Copyright © 2014 Angelo T Scotti, M.D.
All rights reserved.

ISBN: 1499339682
ISBN 13: 9781499339680
Library of Congress Control Number: 2014908455
CreateSpace Independent Publishing Platform
North Charleston, South Carolina

The advice, concepts and recommendations in this book are not intended as a substitute for medical advice from a professionally trained and/or licensed practitioner. You should consult with your physician before starting this or any other dietary plan. The author disclaims any liability arising directly or indirectly from the use of this publication.

THE DR. SCOTTI DIET

TABLE OF CONTENTS

Chapter 1

WHY THIS DIET WILL

WORK FOR YOU

In seeing well over 100,000 patients in 42 years as a practicing physician, I have learned three things without question: most people want to lose weight, few people actually do, and those who do almost never keep the weight off. I witnessed thousands of patients make the attempt, only to fail. Some of them failed quickly. Others met with initial success, then gradually put the weight back on, often gaining more than they'd ·lost.

When I saw the sadness in the eyes of my patients as they struggled with their weight, I remembered why I became a doctor in the first place. It is because when I was just a boy of 7 years old, doctors saved my mother's life at a T.B. clinic. I missed her dearly and as I closed my eyes countless times in the two years she was away from us, I imagined those doctors helping her. So it was *then* I knew *exactly* what I wanted to do. I wanted to help others, just as those in the clinic helped my mom.

Through trial and error and more than a few mistakes, I crafted a plan that allowed my patients to not only lose weight, but also to keep that weight off.

Permanently.

Because when my patients lose weight and keep it off, they are not only happier and have a much more positive self-image, but are also healthier and at a decreased risk of both cancer and heart disease.

I am well aware that many people diet so they will feel more attractive and not because they want to become healthier. But I am happy I have been able to harness my patients' desires to feel more attractive, and use it as a tool to propel them on the path to becoming more healthy, regardless of their underlying motivations.

In the following pages, I lay out The Dr. Scotti Diet. Several hundred of my patients have lost, collectively, thousands of pounds using this diet. The vast majority of whom, because of the personalized nature of the diet and the ease at which it can be self-administered, have been able to keep the weight off for the long-term.

I feel the diet has been honed to the point that I am ready to share it with the world. And I hope you will join those who have already experienced victory in their battle against those extra pounds.

The Founding Principles of The Dr. Scotti Diet

I believe much of the success my patients have had with this diet is a direct result of the following engines that form the core concepts of the plan. In order for a diet to be successful, it must not only work in theory, but must also be easy and agreeable enough to stick with over the long-term. Failure to adhere to these ideals, in my opinion, is one of the major reasons that although there are over 400 verified diets that currently exist, over 98% of dieters fail to lose weight or keep their loss off. This is incredible to me, and as a direct result, The Dr. Scotti Diet has been built upon a foundation of five basic principles:

1. Individuality: Weight Gaining Foods, Weight Neutral Foods, and Weight Losing Foods. Each of us has a unique genetic finger-print that causes us to metabolize various foods in different ways. As a result of the way our individual bodies process and store the energy from the things we eat, there are three overall classes of foods that apply to each of us: Weight Gaining Foods, Weight Neutral Foods, and Weight Losing Foods. As you may imagine, Weight Gaining Foods are those that cause you, as an individual, to put on weight. What may be a Weight Gaining Food for you, may be a Weight Neutral Food for someone else, or even a Weight Losing Food for someone who is lucky enough to have a naturally high metabolism.

2. Experimentation: Finding What Works for You. One of the reasons this diet has been successful is that it stems from the concept of "personalized trial and error". You will experiment daily with new foods, discovering which cause you to gain or lose weight. It is not based on a rigid set of one-size-fits-all rules. Instead, it is more flexible and realistic.

3. Sustainability: There Are No Forbidden Foods on The Dr. Scotti Diet. Another reason for the success of this diet is there are no foods that are *strictly* forbidden. As you work your way through the simple stages of the diet, which we will discuss shortly, all foods you eat will be classified into one of the three categories listed above. As a result, you will know *exactly* which foods will cause you to gain weight. Therefore, if you choose to eat these foods, you will be aware that you will have to counter that weight gain with some sort of Balancing Activity. Thus, Weight Gaining foods are not forbidden, but you must be sure the Balancing Activity is of the adequate amount in order to compensate. I believe the fact that nothing is strictly forbidden drastically increases the chances of the dieter actually sticking with the diet.

4. Balancing Activities: Tools to Help You Sustain Your Target Weight. These are activities and techniques that you can use during your long-term target weight maintenance. They can be used to help reduce your weight after you have consumed a Weight Gaining Food. Balancing Activities are the keys to your long-term success. They include: Glycemic Index substitution, matching foods, increased physical activity, decreased portion size, fasting, and abstinence.

5. The Power of Empirical Evidence: Basing the Diet on Real Life. In medicine, the most enduring of concepts are those that are based on direct observation and experimentation. This is what we call *empirical evidence*. This concept has always appealed to me because I believe if something is observed over and over again across a range of patients and situations, there is a high likelihood that what has been observed, reflects the truth. As a result, The Dr. Scotti Diet was formed through direct observation of my patients, and more importantly *how they actually live their lives*. Not on theories on how they should live their lives, nor my rules, but on parameters through which they actually live their lives, lose weight, and keep it off. Therefore, the techniques described in the following pages have been tested on the proving grounds, through trial and error, of my patients lives, and of course, on their scales. And, thankfully, I've seen entire families lose weight on this diet. As one patient, a husband and father of two put it, "No one is starving or unhappy. And the food tastes great. And we all look great and feel great."

A Simple Overview of The Dr. Scotti Diet

The Dr. Scotti Diet consists of four simple stages through which you will pass. The first stage is designed to get you to what is called your Target Weight, or simply, the weight you would like to reach. Achieving *and* maintaining this weight are the objectives of The Dr. Scotti Diet. Once you have reached your Target Weight at the end of Stage One, you will pass through Stages Two, Three, and Four, at which time you will be applying the processes of trial and error as you learn which foods are Weight Gaining, Neutral, and Losing Foods for your unique metabolic makeup.

Additionally, the diet consists of a daily routine in which you will weigh yourself each morning just after waking up and using the bathroom, and then record your weight on a simple worksheet called The Food Facts Journal. You will also use this journal to plan and select the foods you will eat, and classify those foods, along with recording other important information.

Lastly, as you discover which are your Weight Gaining Foods, you will employ a Balancing

Activity in order to counteract the weight gain. The interaction between the Balancing Activities and your Weight Gaining Foods are the key to your long-term success of maintaining your Target Weight.

The four stages of The Dr. Scotti Diet are as follows:

1. Stage One: Unlimited Lean Protein and Vegetables. In the initial stage, you will eat only lean proteins and vegetables. Eat all you want. There are no restrictions on portion size or method of preparation. Try to eat at least five vegetables per day in addition to your lean proteins. The only vegetable that should be avoided in this stage are white potatoes. Stage One is complete when you have reached your initial Target Weight, or if you prefer, you may choose to elect another lower Target Weight, and continue with Stage One until you reach it, then move on to Stage Two. Examples of healthy lean proteins include: skinless white chicken or turkey, fish, eggs, soy, non-fat cheese, non-fat cottage cheese, non-fat plain yogurt, beans, and legumes.

2. Stage Two: Finding Friendly Fruits. This stage is the first of the "trial and error" stages, where you will begin to uncover which are your Weight Gaining, Neutral, and Losing Foods. This stage pertains to fruits. You will continue to eat the lean proteins and vegetables from Stage

One, but will now add a single fruit each day, in the amount of one handful. This is defined by the amount of fruit you can hold in one open hand. (We will discuss the measurement of the amount of all foods in more detail in chapter two). The following morning, you will observe the effect fruit has had on your weight. Stage Two is complete when you have identified at least five fruits that are either Weight Losing or Weight Neutral Foods.

3. Stage Three: Adding Grains. This stage is similar to the fruit stage, except you will now be adding one new grain food per day. You will continue to eat the lean proteins and vegetables from Stage One and the fruits from Stage Two, but you will now add foods such as whole-grain bread, sourdough bread, brown rice, and whole wheat pasta. Add foods one at a time, and again in the amount of one handful (one slice for bread). You will observe which are Weight Gaining, Weight Losing, and Weight Neutral Foods. This stage is complete when you have identified several Weight Neutral or Losing grains. There is not a specific number, as this will vary widely from person to person. The key is to have found enough foods collectively by the end of this stage to where you feel you have an abundant variety in what you are eating each day. This will help you as you enter Stage Four, where it is most likely you will encounter some of the more "dangerous" foods.

4. Stage Four: Adding Everything Else.

In this stage, you will continue to eat all the foods from the first three stages, but you will add one new food of *any type* each day. This is the stage where you may add pizza, chocolate, ice cream, cupcakes, cookies, alcohol, or anything else you desire. Again, you will identify which are the weight gaining foods for you, and then choose to not eat them or to eat a limited amount of them and to counter the weight gain with a Balancing Activity. This stage concludes when you have classified all the foods you wish to eat. After that point, you may choose a new, lower Target Weight and repeat the entire four-stage process, or you may choose to maintain your current target weight, using your Food Classifications and Balancing Activities as the foundation of your long-term weight maintenance.

<u>An Introduction to The Balancing Activities</u>

One of the keys to the long-term success of being able to maintain your Target Weight is the interaction between your Weight Gaining Foods and Balancing Activities. These are activities designed to help "balance" the weight gain you will experience as you inevitably, at times during your long-term weight maintenance, choose to eat Weight Gaining Foods. I have found it unrealistic to expect patients will no longer eat any Weight Gaining Foods ever again, so I thought it wise to indentify techniques that would help them. The techniques below will be discussed at greater length in chapters three and four, but I want to introduce them here to get you thinking about them. As stated earlier, I consider these techniques to be realistic, as they are based upon the observations of how my patients actually live their lives. Keep in mind everyone is unique, and the techniques are easily applied by some people and yet can be more difficult for others. I have listed the techniques by rank, in order of effectiveness, combined with ease of application and popularity:

1. Glycemic Index Substitution: This simply means substituting a food that is otherwise similar but has a lower Glycemic Index (G.I.) than another food. Glycemic Index is a popular food ranking system that measures a food based upon its effect on blood-sugar levels. An example of G.I. Substitution would be to purchase and eat whole wheat angel hair pasta instead of regular white penne pasta.

2. Matching Foods: This is defined as matching a Weight Gaining Food with a Weight Losing Food. For instance, if you choose to eat a chocolate ice cream cone, you can then match that with another Weight Losing Food that day.

3. Increased Physical Activity for a Day: This is defined by increasing your physical activity the day you eat the Weight Gaining Food, the next day, or soon after. As will be discussed in chapter five, this does not necessarily mean strenuous physical exercise. A leisurely activity such as walking can suffice.

4. Smaller Portion Size: This is simply reducing the portion sizes of other foods you consume in a day, in order to counter a Weight Gaining Food. It is similar to Matching Foods, but instead of matching one food with another, you eat less of both. For instance, if you want to eat chocolate, you eat one or two squares of that luscious chocolate instead of the entire bar, and then also eat smaller portions of your other foods for the day.

5. Fasting: This is defined as not eating anything for a certain amount of time, which we will discuss later, in order to let your body "make up" for the fact that you have eaten a Weight Gaining Food.

6. Abstinence: This is the least popular of all techniques, but unfortunately, also one of the most effective. This is defined as simply no longer eating a specific Weight Gaining Food. Some people find that, barring a drastic increase in physical exercise, they cannot eat certain foods without gaining weight. This is discussed in greater detail in chapter three.

Processing and Storing Energy: Weight Gaining, Neutral, and Losing Foods

I would like to explain—briefly and without getting too technical—how our bodies metabolize foods, and why one food can be Weight Gaining for one person and Weight Neutral for someone else.

When we eat, our bodies convert the food to a type of sugar called glucose. Then, one of three things can happen, depending on a number of factors:

1. The sugar is burned quickly and used as energy immediately.

2. The sugar is stored in the liver for use in the near future.

3. The sugar is stored as fat for use as energy in the long-term.

Some of the factors that determine which of these three things happen are: our level of physical activity, our genetic metabolism (how quickly we burn or absorb these sugars), how quickly food passes through our gut (the more slowly the food passes through, the more of it is absorbed and converted to sugar), how sensitive our unique body is to a chemical called insulin that allows sugar to enter cells, and other factors.

Just as one medication can save a patient's life who is suffering from a certain illness, it can have no effect on another person suffering from that same illness, or potentially kill yet another patient who happens to be highly allergic to that medication. Each person's unique genetic individuality causes their body to interact in a certain way to different things, whether it is medication, food, sunlight, or the weather. This is why one food can be Weight Gaining for me, but Weight Neutral for you.

Tools

In addition to the information contained in this book, all you will need is a working scale upon which you can weigh yourself each morning, a notebook (either paper or digital, whichever you are more likely to use) that you will designate as your Food Facts Journal, and access to the internet, so you can search for the Glycemic Index of your favorite foods, and also for recipes that will keep you on track.

Chapter 2

THE DR. SCOTTI DIET

Before beginning The Dr. Scotti Diet you must prepare yourself, your family, and your kitchen. You will also need your scale and journal. The first step in the process is to choose your initial Target Weight.

Picking Your Initial Target Weight

The Dr. Scotti Diet is *your* plan and only *you* can decide a target goal. You can, however, change your target as you proceed, depending on how you respond, how you look, how you feel, and your feedback from others who care for you. But you must pick a target.

The great majority of my patients initially choose an unrealistic target weight based on their high school graduation weight, their wedding day, their weight before their first child, or simply what they would like to weigh. Most do not reach such goals, but a few actually do so.

My usual suggestion is to delay your actual *final* weight goal until you have been on your diet for a number of weeks. Choose a reasonable starting goal as a first step while at Stages One and Two. A reasonable and achievable first goal is 5 to 10% of your weight at that point. Do not begin Stage Four until you have reached a 10% loss from your original weight and maintained that for at least one month.

If you lose weight during Stages One through Three, but fail to hit the 10% mark and simply plateau, take a critical look at your naked body in the mirror. Then take a look with your clothes on, and then take a moment to look only at your face. I know this may seem odd at first. But I have come to notice an interesting phenomenon with many of my patients: when comparing their body to their face while looking in the mirror, there is a clear difference in weights at which they believe they look best.

I also have patients who have different target weights depending on the season. They choose to gain a bit in winter to look younger and healthier with a slightly fuller face, while their bulky clothes hide their modest weight gain. Then, in summer, they trim down.

Your Target Weight can always be adjusted to meet your changing needs and desires. But it is a required tool in The Dr. Scotti Diet. So, pick your target and shoot for it!

Weighing Yourself Daily

On The Dr. Scotti Diet, each day begins with a trip to the scale. As soon as you get up in the morning, your first stop is the bathroom to empty your bladder. Every day, step on the scale while naked, weigh yourself, and record your weight. Your food choices will be determined by this daily ritual.

Beginning The Dr. Scotti Diet

Now that you have chosen a Target Weight, you will empty your cupboard of food by eating it or giving it away so you can start with a clean slate. Make a list of foods to purchase containing only low fat proteins and vegetables, except white potatoes. Eat a large meal of whatever you want before going grocery shopping. At the store buy only those foods on your list. All diets begin at the grocery store! I will discuss more on how to successfully shop in chapter eight.

Remember: each day begins with your weigh-in, which you will record in a journal.

Stage One: Initial Weight Loss

The objective of Stage One is direct weight loss. This is the stage that will allow you to achieve your initial Target Weight, while Stages Two through Four will be more focused on maintaining that weight.

During Stage One, you will eat only vegetables and low fat proteins. You should eat at least five different vegetables each day, and all the low fat proteins you would like. As I said before, examples of healthy lean proteins include: skinless white chicken or turkey, fish, eggs, soy, nonfat cheese, non-fat cottage cheese, non-fat plain yogurt, beans, and legumes.

Eat as much as you desire of each; do not allow yourself to be hungry. Being full and satiated is the best defense against eating the wrong foods.

Upon reaching your initial Target Weight, decide whether or not you are satisfied with this weight or want to lose more.

If you decide to pick a new, lower, Target Weight at this point, you can extend Stage One and continue the low fat proteins and vegetables for as long as you wish. Once satisfied with your weight loss, you are ready for Stage Two and the addition of fruit.

Over the years that I have been prescribing this diet, I have come to understand the difficulties encountered by patients during Stage One. Patients never hesitate to tell me things they struggle with. These include lack of variety, craving for their favorite (weight gaining) foods, dislike of all the foods on the list, and difficulty overcoming their resistance to change.

One observation I have made is that for many patients, a few days of weight loss often helps because they begin to see the results of their efforts, and this is encouraging for them.

Those who are ultimately successful with this diet come to understand that each of the high protein, low fat foods can be prepared in many different ways. This provides them with the variety they are craving, and allows them to stick with it long enough to start seeing major results, which then carries them further along in the process.

For example, eggs can be scrambled, fried, poached, hardboiled, soft boiled, and mixed with vegetables in an omelet. White meat chicken and turkey can be soaked in vinegar, covered with mustard, or smothered with herbs, pepper, and salt. Condiments, which have little or no calories, such as vinegar, lemon juice, and mustard add flavor and variety to fish and fowl.

Soy products take various forms such as soy milk, soy nuts, tofu, edamame (green vegetable soy beans), soy flower, soy protein powder, and soy yogurt. You can browse soy recipes on the web. Fish can be prepared in many ways including baked, broiled, grilled—all with the use of condiments. One of my favorite dishes are eggs scrambled with salmon, onions, mushrooms, tomatoes, and spinach.

Again, a web search for any given vegetable can provide scores of ways to prepare any you may wish to try. Seaweed is one of the most nutritious foods and a Google search of "seaweed preparation" revealed ideas for various salads, soups, and cooked seaweed. One book on pre-Columbian Indians of New England mentioned an Indian woman who could make over 120 different foods from corn. Therefore, choose a few vegetables and search the web.

While the main objective of Stage One is weight loss, the objective for Stage Two is maintaining the lower weight while you add non-weight gaining fruit.

5 Ways to Eat 5 Vegetables Each Day

1. Raw: Cut up 4 vegetables and use Hummus as a dip, non-fat yogurt could also be used or a non-fat cheese dip.

2. Vegetable Soup: cook yourself, take out at a restaurant, or buy it canned.

3. Roasted vegetables.

4. Steamed vegetables with lemon, ginger, and herb dressing (at Stage Four Olive Oil dressing)

5. Blend 5 vegetables and drink.

Stage Two: Finding Friendly Fruits

In Stage Two, you will add one handful of fruit to your diet each day, in addition to your five vegetables and various low fat proteins foods you ate in Stage One. If your weight does not increase the next day, continue with that fruit and add one handful of a different fruit on day two. Continue the process until you are eating five different fruits each day.

Remember, you must weigh yourself each morning and record your weight in your journal.

If your weight increases at all after adding a new fruit, cross that fruit off your list and try a different one. By trial and error you should be able to add five fruits to your diet. If most of the fruits you try cause weight gain, check the Glycemic Index on fruits and try those that have a lower Glycemic Index than the ones you had to reject.

If you still cannot come up with five non-weight gaining fruits, eat only those which were acceptable and add one new vegetable each day to make a total of ten fruits and vegetables per day.

Although Stage Two is primarily a weight maintenance stage, many people actually lose weight by choosing fruits from their Weight Losing list. Continue Stage Two for as long as you desire since a diet of fruits, vegetables, and low fat protein is healthy as well as energy producing.

The major obstacle some of my patients run into during Stage Two is they can come up with five fruits they enjoy, but finding five that are Weight Neutral or Weight Losing is another thing altogether. The solution is to try your favorite fruits first and if you gain weight, switch to your second most favorite, and so on.

One major aid is to look up the Glycemic Index and begin with those fruits which have the lowest number rating. If you cannot find five fruits which are acceptable by taste and weight criteria, then you can substitute with vegetables.

5 Ways to Eat 5 Fruits Each Day

1. Fruit Salads.

2. Eat single fruits as snacks throughout the day or as trail mix (dried fruit & nuts) once you reach Stage Four.

3. Cook a compost of fruits; this is especially good for those with allergies to raw fruit and or skins.

4. Blend five fruits; you can even mix these with your vegetable blends.

5. Whole grain cereals (once you reach Stage Three) and skim milk, soy milk or (once you reach Stage Four) almond milk, with 5 fruit.

Stage Three: Adding Grains

In Stage Three, you will add one whole grain to your diet each day. Whole grain foods are those that have not been processed to remove the fiber and include whole wheat bread, brown rice, and whole wheat pasta. Check the label to be sure there is no refined grain. These foods are commonly called *starches* and are healthy but can cause weight gain.

Use the same process you did for fruit by adding a handful of bread, pasta, or rice. Weigh yourself the next day and omit any whole grain foods from your diet which result in <u>any</u> weight gain the following morning. Again, use trial and error with the help of the Glycemic Index table in order to help you pick Weight Neutral foods (starches are rarely associated with loss of weight).

Some will find they cannot maintain their weight loss with <u>any</u> starches, but most people can tolerate some without regaining the weight. Stage Three is also a weight maintenance phase with little or no loss of weight for most people.

As I mentioned, adding starches also has the major risk of weight gain, especially if you immediately return to those that caused weight gain in the first place.

Do not go back to those favorites that you know make you gain weight or which clearly do so during your daily weight measurements. Go back to the Glycemic Index list and start with starches with a low G.I. Some people cannot return to starches and still maintain their new lower weight. Skipping the starches completely is one solution. But if you view that as something you cannot reasonably do, other solutions include the Balancing Activities mentioned in Chapter One including extra exercise, periodic fasting, or smaller portions.

Remember: starches are the most common cause of obesity and you must do whatever it takes to deal with them.

Stage Three is complete when you have found a sufficient number of Weight Neutral or Losing grains, or you have exhausted the options and have found <u>all</u> grains are Weight Gaining Foods for you, and thus must be eliminated from your diet.

Stage Four: Adding Everything Else

During Stage Four, the final stage, you will add <u>any</u> foods of your choice, simply to make your daily eating habits satisfying enough to keep you from returning to your old ways—which made you over-weight in the first place. Add foods just as you did with fruits and grains, one handful of each new food per day while monitoring with daily weigh-ins.

Some of your favorites may be Weight Neutral, and those should remain part of your diet if you still enjoy them. Unfortunately, others will cause weight gain and *how* you deal with those foods is a critical factor in your success. The safe and simple solution of these fat-causing favorites is to omit them completely.

However, if there are foods you enjoy so much you will eat them even though they cause weight gain when merely sampled, there are ways to counteract this effect. Just as they are with Stage Three, the Balancing Activities are a critical tool for the success of your long-term weight man-agement in Stage Four.

For instance, you may occasionally indulge in these fattening choices by choosing the form of that food (e.g. pizza) with the lowest Glycemic Index. Check the G.I. chart for pizza to see which have the lowest G.I. Do the same with any favor-ite candidates.

Smaller portions, limiting the amount you prepare or buy, and using smaller plates may all be helpful. Try trading some other relatively high G.I. foods (e.g. fruit or bread) for a vegetable in order to save some calories. Fasting with a liquid diet the day after you indulge also works.

For those who are willing to exercise, you can pick up the pace and burn more calories the day before, the day of, or the day after an indulgence. Some of my patients have maintained their well-earned weight loss by combining some of the techniques mentioned. For example, they will increase their physical activity for a few days, indulge and then go on liquid diet the day after indulging. The typical day for indulging tends to be Saturday or Sunday.

If you cannot or will not do what it takes to safely indulge the favorite foods that cause weight gain, you have to face yourself and make some decisions. Can you be more successful with a different favorite food? If not, are the few minutes of pleasure you experience while indulging worth the price you will pay?

Look at yourself in the mirror, and then look at a picture of you before beginning your diet. If that doesn't help you decide what to do, there is one last hope. Eat a great quantity of that sinful food in one day and nothing else that day. Gorging may cure you of the craving. The next day go back to where you left off.

In order to maintain your targeted lower weight you must weigh yourself daily, and eat at least five vegetables and some low fat protein <u>before</u> you indulge in fruits, grains (starches), and other potentially fattening foods. Don't dine out until you reach your Target Weight and only do so if you can maintain your diet.

There are usually reasonable choices available at most restaurants and diners as well as some fast food places. But some of the fast food restaurants have <u>no</u> reasonable choices for those who do not choose to be fat. Check the menu online <u>before</u> you go.

Once you have your diet under control and you feel confident you can control your weight, avoid being hungry by filling up on your weight loss foods and by avoiding foods with a high Glycemic Index (such as white bread, rice, pasta, etc.) which increase your insulin levels, make you crave starches, and result in loss of control over your diet. At this point you can even pick a new, lower target weight and go for it.

If you "fall off the wagon," lose control of your diet, and begin packing on the adipose tissue, <u>do</u> <u>not </u>stop your daily weigh-ins. Just eat up all of the wrong foods you brought home, don't go back to the store until you are out of these fatteners, and start Stage One over again. Be sure to take pictures of yourself at your fattest and at your lowest weight, print them out, and stick them on your refrigerator. Smile in the skinny one and frown for the fat picture.

One last warning: avoid fats and starches (high Glycemic grains) in the same meal. That combo is a <u>sure</u> weight gainer. Some examples are pizza (dough and cheese), pasta with meatballs or sausages, sandwiches with meat and/or cheese, a cheeseburger (fatty ground beef and cheese, plus bread), a peanut butter and jelly sandwich, pie and ice cream, and most items at fast food restaurants.

As I stated before, Stage Four can be the most dangerous of them all because people tend to return to their previous eating habits. You cannot add all of your old favorites at previous quantities and expect to maintain your new lower weight.

The best solution I have observed was severely limiting or omitting any foods that result in weight gain. *Don't buy them, don't go where they are served, don't visit people who will urge you to eat them.*

By the time you have progressed from Stages One to Three and lost considerable weight, consider how you look, how you feel about yourself, and how others see you before you go back to your old way of eating.

Your Daily Diary

You must routinely weigh yourself each morning and record that weight in order for this diet to be successful. My favorite method of recording is a sheet with columns to record the data, your morning weigh-ins, the added food type, and any weight changes. Another use for the diary is to determine whether or not symptoms arrive or are relieved when you add or subtract specific foods.

One example would be allergies manifested by hives, a rash, itching, or abdominal pain when you ingest a food you are allergic to. Another could be simply food intolerance, such as feeling ill with certain foods. One dramatic situation is gluten sensitivity (Celiac disease), where wheat and other grain containing foods can cause diarrhea, rashes, joint pain, and various other symptoms. If you notice an apparent correlation of a specific food with symptoms, check with your physician for help in determining a cause.

It's not uncommon for patients on the diet to find relief from symptoms that have bothered them for years, only to have the symptoms return when the patient restarts the offending food. Your daily diary can help make this apparent. Following is an example of the format many of my patients have successfully used.

Date	Weight	New Food Added Day Before	Weight Change	Notes or Symptom
2/15	139	Piece of Pizza	+ 1 pound	Abdominal Pain. Pizza is a Weight Gaining Food for me.
2/16	138	None (since gained one pound, decided not to try new food)	- 1 pound	No more pain.
2/17	138	Almonds (handful)	None	Almonds are Weight Neutral for me.
2/18	137	Cheeseburger	+1 pound	Cheeseburgers are a Weight Gaining food for me.

Long-Term Maintenance

The Dr. Scotti Diet is a plan for lifelong weight control, but it is not unchangeable. Foods can be added or removed according to your changing tastes, weight, and life events. As more information becomes available concerning the benefits and risks of various foods, feel free to make changes. The one thing that does not change is your Dr. Scotti Diet approach to weight control.

Daily weight-ins are a must in order to monitor your responses to eating. When you add a new food, start with a handful and note the effect on your weight the next day. Also, note any changes when you discontinue specific foods. Continue to rely on your Balancing Activities as they are key to long-term weight maintenance.

If your weight begins to increase with no apparent change in how you eat, you will need to diagnose the causes. Determine whether or not you have changed the amount of your physical activity, whether or not there have been changes in medications, and whether or not the quantity of what you eat has increased. A visit to your physician can help determine if a medical condition such as diabetes or underactive thyroid may be a contributing factor. The diagnosis will determine your solution. If none of the previously mentioned factors explain your weight gain, it may simply be a change in your metabolism.

In any case, part of the solution is to restart your diet at Stage One, eating low-fat proteins and vegetables, and proceed as you did originally. It almost always works, even if you cannot pinpoint the causes of you unexpected weight gain.

Chapter 3

THE GLYCEMIC INDEX

In order for you to be successful at choosing foods for your diet, it is important you understand the concept of the Glycemic Index. But first, I'll start with a simple explanation of a few things that pertain to the Glycemic Index.

Glucose is the sugar our body burns as fuel. Whenever we eat a carbohydrate, glucose is absorbed through our gut and appears in our blood. The body's response to significant rises in blood glucose is to have the pancreas release insulin into the blood. Insulin allows the glucose to enter cells where it will be utilized and metabolized, or burned, as fuel.

Any excess glucose, above the amount necessary to meet immediate energy needs, will enter fat cells and be stored as fat, a future source of energy in the event that food is not available. Certain foods are slowly absorbed resulting in little or no rise in blood glucose levels; fat and protein are such foods.

Carbohydrates are basically foods that grow in the ground and include vegetables, fruits, and food made from grains. Many foods are combinations of carbohydrates, fat and/or protein, and therefore result in varying and non-predictable associated blood glucose levels. Foods that cause marked and rapid rises in blood glucose tend to cause weight gain.

Blood glucose levels were tested after the ingestion of various carbohydrates (vegetables, fruits, and grains) and it was determined these foods can be *graded* by their effect on those levels. **A grading system from 1 to 100 was developed.** Those foods resulting in small rises in glucose have a lower rating than those causing rapid and high blood glucose levels. **This rating number is called the Glycemic Index (G.I.) of that carbohydrate.**

While there are some variations between individuals, foods with the lowest G.I. are much less likely to cause weight gain than those with a high G.I. At the end of this chapter are lists of carbohydrates with their G.I. levels. In general when attempting to lose weight it is beneficial to choose those foods which have lower G.I. levels. Animal products such as meat have a G.I. level of approximately zero.

The G.I. is helpful when choosing fruits and grains in Stages Two and Three of your diet. This is especially true if you observe a gain in weight the morning after adding a new fruit or grain food. When that occurs simply refer to the G.I. chart for the value of the food and substitute a food with a lower G.I. level.

Keep repeating this process until you find the fruit or grain which is associated with weight loss (a Weight Losing food for you) or at least no change in weight (a Weight Neutral food for you). In Stage Four of your diet the G.I. of complex foods is even more important when choosing your favorite foods while still maintaining your well-earned weight loss.

Carbohydrates are often referred to as complex or simple. Complex carbohydrates are those which have not been altered in any way, presenting just as they grow. Any vegetable or fruit is a complex carbohydrate containing absorbable sugars such as sucrose as well as non-absorbable cellulose, which is better known as fiber. Complex carbohydrates tend to be absorbed slowly and as a result have relatively low G.I. values.

Simple carbohydrates usually refer to grains which have been processed. The bran, cellulose and other difficult to absorb parts have been removed and what is left are simple carbohydrates which are quickly and easily absorbed and converted to glucose in your blood. These simple carbs taste sweet, stimulate insulin secretion, and create hunger and cravings for more of the same. Needless to say, they tend to have high G.I. levels and their ingestion often results in weight gain.

Incidentally, the substance removed in the process which converts complex to simple carbohydrates are often quite nutritious, containing fiber and many beneficial substances which are no longer present in the simple carbs.

Examples of complex grains would include brown rice, whole wheat bread and cereals, and other whole grain bread and pasta. White bread, pancakes from white flour, and white rice and pasta made from "refined flour" are all simple carbs and have relatively high G.I. levels.

It is important to realize each person is unique and while the Glycemic Index can be very helpful in choosing carbs that help you lose weight, it is only a guide. The only real personal test for any food is the morning weigh-in after adding that carb. A single carbohydrate food may be Weight Losing for one person, Weight Neutral for another, and Weight Gaining for someone else, no matter what the table lists as that food's G.I.

Below is a list of some commonly consumed fruits, breads, and cereals, grouped by their G.I. rating (low, medium, and high). To find the G.I. rating for foods not listed below, simply search the Internet using the name of the food and search terms "G.I. rating".

FRUITS

Low

Apples (fresh) - 38
Apples (dried) - 29
Apricots (dried) - 31
Bananas - 52
Blackberries - 25
Blueberries - 25
Canned fruit cocktail - 54
Cherries - 25
Grapefruit - 25
Grapes - 53
Kiwi - 53
Mango - 51
Oranges - 42
Peaches (fresh) - 42
Peaches (in natural juice) - 45
Pears (fresh) - 38
Pears (in natural juice) - 44
Plums - 39
Prunes (pitted) - 29
Raspberries - 40
Strawberries - 40

Medium

Cantaloupe - 67
Cherries (dark) - 63

Cranberries (sweetened) - 64
Figs (dried) - 61
Fruit juices - 55
Papaya - 56
Peaches (in light syrup) - 58
Pineapple - 66
Raisins - 64

High

Dates (pitted) - 100±
Watermelon - 72±

CEREALS

Low

All Bran®, Kellogg's® - 34
All Bran Fruit and Oats®, Kellogg's® - 39
Frosted Flakes®, Kellogg's® - 55
Muesli - Gluten Free - 39 to 54
Oatmeal - Regular Old Fashioned Rolled Oats - 51
Oatmeal - Steel Cut - 52
Rice Bran -19

Medium

Mini Wheat®, Whole Grain, Kellogg's® - 58
Nutri-Grain®, Kellogg's® - 66

Oat Bran Puffed Buckwheat - 65
Rolled Oats, raw - 59
Special K®, Kellogg's® - 59

High

Cheerios®, General Mills® - 77
CoCo Pops®, Kellogg's® - 77
Corn Flakes®, Kellogg's® - 77
Corn Pops®, Kellogg's® - 77
Fruit Loops®, Kellogg's® - 69
Honey Smacks®, Kellogg's® - 71
Mini Wheat®, Kellogg's® - 72
Raisin Bran®, Kellogg's® - 73
Rice Krispies®, Kellogg's® - 82
Shredded Wheat®, Post® - 75

BREADS

Low

Multigrain 9-Grain bread - 43
Pumpernickel - 50
Seeded Rye - 51
Sour Dough Rye - 48
Sour Dough Wheat - 54
Soy and Linseed - 36
Spelt Multigrain - 54
Whole Grain Raisin - 44

Medium

Multigrain Sandwich - 65
Stone Ground Whole Wheat - 59
White Hamburger Bun - 59
White Pita - 57

High

Black Rye - 76
Dark Rye - 86
Gluten Free Multigrain - 79
Kaiser Roll - 73
Lebanese White - 75
Regular Sliced White - 71
White Bagel - 72
White Sandwich - 70
White Wonder - 80
Whole Wheat Enriched Wheat Flour - 70

Chapter 4

BEHAVIOR

One of the key factors in the success of my patients who have lost large amounts of weight with The Dr. Scotti Diet is their ability, willingness, and commitment to alter their behavior. In order to change the way we eat, we must overcome the innate resistance to change the behaviors we've had for most of our lives.

Short of moving to a new cultural area, permanent and drastic changes in eating behavior are rare. Before even attempting to change your eating plan, you must be convinced the new plan can work for you. Belief is key. This occurred to me when I realized that those who participated in religious rituals such as fasting were able to do so because of their deep conviction and dedication to their beliefs.

Belief is a powerfully motivating factor. Most of my patients who have tried the diet have lost significant weight during the first week. That resulted in the first psychological factor necessary—belief in the plan.

The next necessary factor is the desire to lose weight. In my experience, that desire is greatest when a significant life event is upcoming, such as a wedding or reunion. If you are someone who is not easily self-motivated, it is reasonable to pick such an event as your reason for trying the plan. It is also a good time to choose a Target Weight.

Next comes commitment, once you believe the plan can work for you and you have a good reason to try. That commitment includes a resolve to change your eating habits from scratch, almost like an infant being weaned off the breast and introduced to food.

In addition to belief, desire, and commitment you must identify barriers to your success so you can deal with any factors that may undermine your weight reduction plan. Barriers may include other people, even family members, especially those who live with you. Other barriers include: availability of inappropriate food at work, while traveling, at some social engagements, when eating out, and food shopping without a list, especially when you are hungry.

None of the barriers are insurmountable, but it is best to avoid those you are able to, especially during the early stages of your diet. Those that are unavoidable, such as family, can be dealt with by having everyone in the house on their own diet at the same time. I have had a number of families use this approach successfully, especially when most members are overweight, as they often are.

One of the most imposing barriers tends to be lack of self-discipline. Without some planned, reliable disciplinary force, no dietary or other life changes will ever take place. For those with self-discipline, simply the decision to understand and implement the diet is often enough. For the rest some form of external discipline may be required.

External discipline usually means assigning a person other than you to make the food shopping list and do the actual shopping. That person needs to be disciplined, unyielding, reliable, and honest. It helps if the responsible disciplinarian chooses to participate in his or her own diet at the same time.

One of the most detrimental barriers can be a "friend" who does not want to see you lose weight. They can easily be identified by their insistence that you eat something you should not or their disapproval of your plans to change the way you eat. Sometimes that crippling person is a family member.

The solutions to identified barriers to your success are dependent on your unique situations in life, your philosophy, imagination, and your resolve. But each barrier must be recognized before a solution can be sought. One direct approach is to begin the diet as outlined in chapter two, keep a notebook listing deviations from the plan, note the reason for deviations, then construct a written solution to each and try again.

When I explain the diet to a patient and give them a printed copy, their immediate reaction tells me whether or not they will make an attempt. The most frequent initial reaction for those patients who are ultimately successful is their full attention once they hear about the fact that the diet is unique to each person and how it works.

On the other hand, those patients who do not even glance at the printout, neatly fold it up and place it in their pocket, have already communicated their intention. Not one of such patients have ever tried the diet or returned to the office at a lower weight. When a patient is not motivated, I know the timing is not right.

Many religions require fasting at certain times and forbid specific foods. It is impressive to observe religious patients adhere to the limits imposed by their beliefs. I have witnessed an almost religious adherence to the diet once a patient is convinced, by their daily weigh-ins that they are losing weight. Motivation is stimulated by successful weight loss.

One major psychological aid is to anticipate the time when you will be able to control your weight while still eating foods you enjoy that keep you satiated. Do not ruminate about foods you love that you believe will be forbidden; there are no forbidden foods on your diet.

Keep in mind your diet is a systematic way to identify foods that will result in weight gain, so you can make an informed choice regarding how to deal with those foods. Your goal is to have a satisfying way to eat while still maintaining control over your weight. Additionally, you can create an eating plan that also keeps you healthy.

Most people who want to lose weight are motivated by appearance, since they believe they will be more attractive at a lower weight. However, being healthier also adds to your appearance so you can create a personal eating plan which keeps you full, lean, and good looking—all of which will add to your happiness and self-satisfaction.

Chapter 5

PHYSICAL ACTIVITY

Exercise is not necessary for weight loss. With few exceptions, such as marathon runners, triathlon athletes, and long distance bikers, physical activity alone is not sufficient for weight loss. Food intake is the most important factor when trying to slim down.

Physical activity is helpful for looking and feeling better, increasing muscle mass while losing fat, and for overall health as well as longevity. The benefits of being physically active do not require sweating, gym membership, or formal exercise of any kind. Thirty minutes daily of movement is all that is needed.

That body movement can take the form of a physical job, chores that you now pay others to do, an enjoyable hobby such as dancing, kayaking, or hiking, or just walking rather than driving.

An added benefit of making physical activity part of your everyday existence is that it can help you avoid the harmful influence of being sedentary. Sitting more than 3 hours of your waking day undermines any weight loss program. For those who sit at a computer all day, that is very bad news. I now write prescriptions for patients so that provision can be made at work to allow them to stand at their computer. One simple solution is an adjustable food tray used in hospitals when patients take their meals in bed.

If all attempts at incorporating physical activity into your daily routine fail, you need to consider an exercise routine. The simplest approach is walking with a pedometer. Seek to take 10,000 steps per day. A personal gym at home with free weights, treadmill, stationary bike, rowing machine, a mat, chinning bar, and a punching bag was my personal solution. The cost was less than a gym membership as well as more available, more convenient, and much more likely to be utilized. The time spent simply driving to and from a gym is enough for your full daily workout at home.

If you don't enjoy exercise, a TV in your home gym can distract you and help the time go by unnoticed. Your mobile device, or even a DVD player, can offer music and programs for everything from tai chi to yoga to help you use your muscles, while hardly noticing the 30 minutes. The average American spends over 4 hours per day watching TV, sitting the whole time.

Muscles are major calorie burners and the larger the muscle the greater the burning. Your leg and buttock muscles are the biggest and they respond to squats. Combining push-ups, pull ups, chin ups, and sets of core body exercises for your abs is an excellent way to get fit, build muscle, burn a little fat, and develop a body which looks and feels healthy.

Although much is made of aerobic and anaerobic, strengthening and conditioning exercises, the specifics and theory are of little help in the real world of weight control. Simply put, motion helps you burn calories and lose weight and being motionless has the opposite effect. Find ways to turn your motionless time into physical activity. Weight control aside, exercising for 30-90 minutes every day has beneficial effects on longevity, wellbeing, looks, and mood.

Chapter 6

COOKING AT HOME

AND DINING OUT

When you want to lose weight it is best to avoid dining out. The limited choices and multiple temptations can quickly undermine your weight loss plans. The additional social aspects of dining out can, and usually do, result in "cheating" on your diet, especially if you are at Stage One or Two, eating only lean protein, vegetables, and fruits.

Patients often ask, "How can I eat five vegetables and fruits each day?"

My initial response, at least within my own mind, was *just do it*. The question revealed to me how fixed people can be in what and how they eat, that eating is almost a reflex of how they learned to eat as children.

One major advantage to cooking at home is that you have complete control over what you eat and how you eat your food. I can offer what

I have personally done concerning five fruits per day. Each morning I have strawberries, blueberries, blackberries, a banana, and raspberries with a bowl of Cheerios and chocolate almond milk. For those not yet on grains and nuts, enjoy the fruit with skim milk, yogurt, or cottage cheese.

My solution for five vegetables each day is a large bowl of vegetable soup. Each Sunday I make a large pot of vegetable soup with fifteen or more different vegetables and eat it all week. Another favorite of mine is scrambling eggs with five vegetables. If you don't require a lot of variety, eat the same meals every day and if variety is important to you, change the fruits and vegetables. Salads are another easy method of getting both vegetables and fruits.

For those who have little desire to prepare meals, a fast and simple solution is a food blender. Combinations of vegetables, fruits, or both can be put into liquid form for fast consumption. If time during the week is limited, soups and blended foods can be made in large quantities on a weekend and frozen for use during the busy week.

If cooking is something you enjoy, The Dr. Scotti Diet offers opportunities to be creative by preparing delicious traditional meals within the parameters of your plan. You can explore low Glycemic foods which you like and low calorie condiments and spices such as herbs, vinegar, lemon juice, spices, and mustard. Avoid frying, but other cooking methods such as roasting, grilling, and microwaving are reasonable choices.

Dining out is a major challenge during the early development of your diet and is best avoided until you reach your goal weight and have maintained it for at least a few weeks. Once you feel in control of your diet and are not adding new foods, dining out can be done with satisfaction and no damage to your program. For your initial meals out, go to places you are certain have meals on the menu that fit your diet, or a chef who will accept the challenge of your food and preparation perimeters. Once while having dinner in a hotel with an associate, he could find nothing on the menu acceptable to him. To my surprise he had the waitress make a special request to the chef. He asked for a delicious vegetarian dish of the chef's own choosing and received an excellent meal that fit his eating plan.

Traditional ethnic restaurants often have excellent choices that can meet your diet needs. Traditional American restaurants are a bigger challenge, and fast food restaurants are the most difficult of all when attempting to maintain your diet and weight status. I have been on the same diet for many years and can do this successfully in most food establishments, but dining out is never as effective as eating at home.

The alternative to dining out when you cannot be at home is packing your own food. Then you have complete control. A major problem when dining out is portion size, as you usually end up with more food than you would prepare and eat at home. A simple solution is eating 1/3 to ½ of your meal and bringing the rest home. Another useful approach is reviewing menus of the possible restaurants before you go, picking the best place and choosing before you ever leave home.

Although some fast food restaurants are making efforts to provide healthful, weight sensitive food choices, they have a long way to go and the availability of meals that are detrimental to your diet is a temptation that some cannot resist. Test yourself when you feel confident and if your weight is up the day after visiting a specific restaurant, cross it off your list.

The good news is that when you find your perfect version of The Dr. Scotti Diet and have maintained your weight, the lure, taste, and satisfaction you previously experienced from foods that made you fat no longer have the same hold over you.

Chapter 7

ALCOHOL

Many patients begin asking when they can drink alcohol on The Dr. Scotti Diet. The simple answer is after you have reached your target weight, are on lean proteins, vegetables, fruits, and whole grains.

Heavy daily drinkers (three or more alcoholic drinks per day) can lose weight simply by discontinuing alcohol since alcohol has more calories (7) per gram than carbohydrates (4). Some studies have indicated that those who drink one or two drinks per day actually live longer than non-drinkers. However, alcohol can be toxic and should be avoided by alcoholics and limited to no more than ½ of a drink per day for women who are at increased risk of breast cancer.

The reality is that a high percentage of people will not continue on any eating plan that completely excludes alcohol from their diet. For those who want to drink, knowledge concerning the calorie count of various drinks can help them add alcohol to their diet without compromising their hard-won weight loss.

Alcohol can actually be used by some people to decrease hunger. Stress eaters may also profit by the anti-anxiety effects of alcohol. An alcoholic drink can replace dessert with a great saving in calories since light beer, white wine, and champagne are all under 100 calories per drink, which is much lower than most desserts. For example, an ice cream sundae, New York cheesecake, apple crispetti, and chocolate molten cake all have 1,200 or more calories.

Since many social occasions involve alcohol, it is best to avoid them during the developmental periods of your diet, unless you have great self-discipline. Another approach is to be the designated driver.

When you do add alcohol to your diet, take a look at the following chart before you make your choices. More information is available in a pocket-sized bartender's guide which you can purchase.

COMMON ALCOHOLIC BEVERAGES	Ounces	Calories
Budweiser® beer	12.0	145
Bud Light® beer	12.0	110
Miller light® beer	12.0	96
Merlot, red wine	5.0	119
Chardonnay, white wine	5.0	120

Champagne, dry	4.0	105
Champagne, pink	4.0	100
Mike's Hard Lemonade®	11.2	240
Bacardi Silver® drinks	12.0	225
(flavored drinks have		
different calorie counts)		
Bacardi Silver low carb®	12.0	94
(black cherry or		
green apple)		

10 COMMON MIXED DRINKS	Ounces	Calories
1. Martini	2.5	155
2. Mojito	3.5	149
3. Margarita	8.0	371
4. Long Island Iced Tea	8.3	276
5. White Russian (Kahlua® Ready-To-Drink)	8.0	567
6. Mudslide	8.0	559
7. Strawberry Daiquiri	8.0	229
8. Piña Colada	8.0	437
9. Bloody Mary	10.0	124
10. Lemon Drop (low carb)	2.75	125

Chapter 8

SHOPPING FOR FOOD

I can still remember the conversation I had several years ago with one of my patients that illustrated the struggle many go through while shopping at the grocery store. A wife and mother of three children, all of whom were overweight, spoke of the shame and horror she felt as she realized, each time, that she had filled her shopping cart with weight gaining foods. It was a remark she made during our conversation that stuck with me.

"Dr. Scotti, it feels as if I'm helpless when I'm in the store. It feels almost hopeless, really. And then there's the fact that I'm trying to shop for my kids and my husband, and also trying to buy the correct things for myself and my diet at the same time," she explained.

This conversation put me on the alert for other similar struggles that my patients who were on The Dr. Scotti Diet experienced as they went shopping. Just as I had with other aspects of the process, I began asking them questions about their shopping experiences, and listened to stories of their struggles and the techniques they came up with on their own that worked well for them.

Over the years, after speaking with hundreds of my patients about the subject, it became apparent to me that when it comes to grocery shopping while on a diet (any diet), *the battle is won or lost before you leave your home.*

As a result, below are shopping suggestions and lessons I have learned while speaking with patients who have successfully used The Dr. Scotti Diet. For ease of navigation, I have broken the list down into four categories: Before, During, and After Shopping, and While Traveling.

Before Shopping

The two most effective techniques I have seen used by my patients prior to heading off to the food store are:

1. Make a Detailed Shopping List and Mentally Commit to Buying *Only* What Is On That List.

Putting together your shopping list will help you plan properly for staying within the stage-specific parameters of the diet, and will also act as a sort of armor against straying into dangerous waters once you have entered the food store. Making the list will reinforce your commitment to the diet, remind you of which foods you have classified as Weight Gaining, force you to plan sufficient Balancing Activities to counter that weight gain, and also help you to choose delicious and healthy meals in the days after you shop.

When assembling your list, the first step is to refer to which stage of the diet you are currently in. If you are in Stage One, your list will consist of lean proteins and vegetables. To keep things interesting, for instance, you can aim to eat through the entire rainbow of colors when it comes to vegetables, or try some new lean protein you've never had before. Similarly, when you are in Stage Three, you can try experimenting with one of the newly-popular alternative grains such as quinoa, or try a new twist on an old favorite, such as brown-rice pasta.

If you are in Stage Two, Three, or Four, you will be in the "trial and error" phase and will need to decide which single "new" food you will be testing each day in order to classify it. Additionally, as you progress through the stages and have more information, you will begin planning for recipes that call for a number of foods, which you will classify as either Weight Gaining, Neutral, or Losing. Referring to your Food Facts Journal, you should seek to classify your total food purchases so they loosely resemble the following:

- 60% - 70% Weight Losing Foods
- 30% - 40% Weight Neutral Foods
- 5% - 10% Weight Gaining Foods

Over time, I have found the above percentages drastically increase a dieter's chances of sticking with the diet and also of finding success in maintaining their Target Weight over the long-term. By allowing themselves to eat some Weight Gaining Foods, they can control and compartmentalize the foods and/or cravings associated with those foods in a measured manner, and also deal with the accompanying weight gain with a sufficient Balancing Activity.

An additional note about purchasing Weight Gaining Foods is that you should seek to buy the smallest quantity available. Do not buy a one-pound bag of your favorite candy or a container of one dozen cupcakes if all you really need is one. This is especially true if you happen to shop at some of the large wholesale membership discount food warehouses. If you happen to get caught with an especially strong craving while you are shopping at one of these warehouses, it can be easy to end up owning several pounds of your favorite candy, which, for any dieter and because we are all human, can mean disaster.

Once you have assembled your list, take a moment to search for any opportunities to trade known Weight Gaining Foods for those that are Weight Neutral. Additionally, focus on the carbohydrates included on your list, then refer to your Glycemic Index Guide to check if there are any that can be swapped for those that have a lower Glycemic Index.

When assembling their lists, many of my successful patients would select a few healthy meals that sounded delicious to them and that they found to be fairly easy to prepare. Many times these would include savory stir-fries, meals containing fresh fish and vegetables, soups, hearty salads, fruit salads, smoothies, and sandwiches. I would recommend seeking out recipes for those that appeal to you. A quick Google or YouTube search for recipes can make things extremely easy for even the most picky of dieters.

To set yourself up for post-shopping success, I would also recommend that you plan to purchase some foods that are Weight Losing or Neutral Foods that require little or no preparation. These are the types of foods that can be kept in the refrigerator or on the counter, and can be eaten at a moment's notice when the urge to snack comes. Common examples include things such as carrots or celery with hummus, ripe seedless grapes, and freshly cooked, prepared lentil or vegetable soup.

Another relatively common problem my patients came across was they would have to put things on their list for other members of their family who were not participating in the diet. Especially in the first few weeks of the diet, these patients were vulnerable to eating many of the foods their other family members wanted because the foods were easily accessible. The patients then seemed to "blame" their children and partners for their lack of ability to stick to the parameters of the diet. This is an issue you will need to, as one of my patients put it, "think creatively" to overcome. Two examples of successful techniques include shopping for only yourself for the first few weeks, and asking a partner to shop for the those members of the family who are not on the diet, or making the diet a family function and including everyone on the program, as The Dr. Scotti Diet works especially well for overweight families.

2. Eat A Full Meal or A Weight Gaining Food Just Before Leaving For The Store.

Many patients have mentioned (and I think that most of us can certainly agree) that if they head off to the food store on an empty stomach, they are doomed. Eating a full meal prior to leaving for the grocery store is a technique that works well in bolstering one's resolve when it comes to sticking to your shopping list. If this full meal happens to contain some fat, it is even more likely to help the dieter feel satiated as they shop, and thus less likely to fall victim to the tricks supermarkets use (discussed later) to get unsuspecting shoppers to make impulse purchases that will have a detrimental effect on their diet.

One of my patients came up with a bit of an unorthodox technique I thought worth mentioning. She always ate a Weight Gaining Food on purpose before she left for the store. "That way, when I'm there, I not only feel full, but I also feel guilty for eating the Weight Gaining Food. And the guilt helps keep me honest, I guess," she told me. I thought it was interesting because it was so honest and so simple. And when I mentioned the technique to others, with her permission of course, many of them immediately responded positively to it.

3. Other Recommendations for Before You Leave

If you are worried about your ability to only purchase what is on your shopping list, you may want to consider "partnering up" with a friend or relative (preferably someone who is also on The Dr. Scotti Diet), and having them act as a chaperone as you shop. If they are also on the diet, the two (or more) of you can be mutual supporters. Alternatively, if you feel you are not yet ready to shop, you can ask a supportive partner or friend to initially do some of the shopping for you.

Another technique many of my patients found helpful, especially in the initial stages of the diet, was to not bring their children with them when they shopped for food. I know this may not be a viable alternative for many, but I thought it worth mentioning. As many of us know, children are easy targets for the products that have been marketed specifically toward them (and also placed at their eye-level in many of the aisles). They have a tendency to want these things passionately, and this can cause you to lose focus on your mission of sticking to your shopping list. And, obviously, you want to make doing so as hassle-free as possible.

If you are able, I recommend you plan on doing your food shopping at times that are "off-peak" at the grocery stores. Specifically, times to avoid are Sundays, when most folks are buying for their workweek, and also on weekdays after five o' clock, when many other people are shopping for that night's dinner.

Lastly, before you leave, you may want to gather photos on your phone or in your Food Facts Journal to keep you company as you shop. Many of my patients have found that for some reason, photos help remind them of healthy and tasty meals they are going to prepare, or, of the body they will have when they reach their target weight.

While You Are At the Store

Once you arrive at the store, you should constantly be reminding yourself you will buy only what is on the list. This should be your mantra. The plan should be to get in and get out as quickly as possible. You will need to stay focused because there are many things specifically designed to throw you off track.

For instance, in an effort to get you to purchase more products through impulse buys, supermarkets are known to employ the following techniques:

• Making commonly purchased foods (milk, bread, etc.) either difficult to locate or at opposite ends of the store in order to get you to hunt for them.

• Reorganizing the store periodically to confuse you so you must then hunt for things you once knew the location of.

• Grouping "suggested" foods together, that may be from different food groups. (It can be argued this is for shopper convenience, but it is especially worth noting for The Dr. Scotti Dieter, who doesn't want to be fooled.) An example is that display rack of salsa in front of the chips.

• Putting high impulse-buy probability foods at the checkout counter

You must be aware of these tricks and business practices so you will be able to mentally defend against them as you stay focused and remind yourself to buy only what is on your list.

Additionally, if you are Abstaining or using a Balance Activity, I would recommend avoiding any food aisles that do not pertain to you. The marketing of foods to the consumer, through packaging and aisle placement, has become so effective that at times even the most dedicated can falter.

I am not surprised most of my patients have found that when they do stray from their list, it is for an impulse buy of a Weight Gaining Food. As human beings, we are imperfect. The first thing to realize is it can happen to anyone. The second thing to realize is you have choices that can help mitigate some of the damage.

For instance, if you have decided you are going to stray, I would recommend buying the absolute smallest portion of the offending item that you can. Alternatively, check if there are any acceptable substitutes which have a lower Glycemic Index rating. Lastly, you may want to put some of the other foods back, and balance the calories of the Weight Gaining Food against the absence of the other foods.

Returning Home

Once you return home from the store, there are two key elements to setting yourself up for success:

1. Make the Weight Losing and Neutral Foods Easily Accessible. My son Dave once made the observation that he could eat an entire tray of cupcakes in the time it takes to peal an orange. This stuck with me, and so I explored the concept in conversations with my patients. I soon found this technique had merit. As discussed earlier, it is important to ensure the good foods are within a moment's reach, so when the urge comes to snack, those are the ones which are eaten. I would also recommend washing any vegetables, and pre-cooking whatever you can, to further fill your refrigerator with an abundance of easily accessible Weight Losing and Neutral Foods.

2. Keep the Weight Gaining Foods Out of Sight. I also recommend you keep any Weight Gaining Foods off the countertops, and out of the front of the refrigerator and the pantry. Because you purchased these foods with a specific Balancing Activity in mind, and to be eaten on a certain day or after a certain meal, there is no need to tempt yourself to eat them early, or in a larger portion than you originally planned.

When Traveling

Through conversations with my patients and also through my own personal experience, I know it can be much more difficult to stay on track while you are traveling. Once we are knocked out of our routine, where we have our own kitchen to prepare our foods, our familiar restaurants where we already know what we are going to order, and our (sometimes) familiar stores from which we purchase our food, things can become more challenging.

The key is to maintain focus and do what you can to stay on track before you leave. If you have a set itinerary, you can research the menus of the restaurants where you will be staying. If you are lucky, you will be staying at a place that has a kitchen or at least is amenable to preparing simple foods. If not, you will need to stay flex-ible and be aware you will need to try harder to eat the way you wish to eat. Actively maintain a positive mental attitude, and you will soon find yourself sampling new foods or new ways of pre-paring familiar ones.

I'm convinced that, just as it is with shopping regularly at your local store, when it comes to travel and dieting, the battle is won before you even leave home.

Chapter 9

THE 20 HEALTHIEST FOODS

While developing your diet, consider adding some of the healthiest foods to your diet. Since we are all unique individuals there is no such thing as a food that is healthy for everyone. You could be allergic to any food and become sick or die from eating one of the so-called healthiest foods. But barring an allergy, some foods appear to be generally healthier for most people than others.

By healthy foods I mean those which are most likely to provide beneficial substances such as vitamins, minerals, essential amino acids, antioxidants, fiber, and healthy plant fats. The absence of saturated fat, pesticides, and other harmful substances were also considered when choosing the foods.

Certain foods have been associated with decreases in illnesses such as heart disease and cancer while others are known to be associated with increases in these and other illnesses. The associations with illness also influenced the food choices listed here.

I will not discuss the various theories associated with the good and bad correlations or claim there is a cause and effect relationship between food and diseases. It simply makes sense to avoid foods associated with disease and eat those of your liking which have no bad connection or, even better, eat those connected with health benefits.

These twenty superstars make the list because they scored the highest overall when put to the test. I scrutinized hundreds of foods, from lettuce to lollipops, using the following:

- -Vitamins and mineral content
- -Essential Amino Acids content
- -Antioxidants
- -Glycemic Index
- -Fiber quantity
- -Traces of pesticide
- -Omega 3
- -Saturated fat
- -Illness prevention
- -Illness producing

SUPER FOODS

1. **FISH** (wild salmon, wild sardines, rainbow trout)
2. **NUTS** (almonds, pecans, walnuts)
3. **LEAFY GREENS**** (organic spinach, kale, watercress)
4. **EGGS** (free range)

5. **BERRIES** (blueberries, raspberries, strawberries, cherries)
6. **BROCCOLI, CAULIFLOWER, BRUSSELS SPROUTS**
7. **AVOCADO**
8. **ONIONS, GARLIC**
9. **BEANS** (lentils, garbanzo, black)
10. **YOGURT**
11. **OATMEAL**
12. **SEAWEED**
13. **SKIM MILK** (organic)
14. **MUSHROOMS**
15. **OLIVES** (and olive oil)
16. **COCONUTS** (and coconut oil)
17. **HERBS**
18. **MANGOES, POMEGRANATE**
19. **TOMATOES**
20. **ROOT VEGETABLES** (carrots, organic potatoes**, beets)

** High incidence of pesticide. For these foods, I recommend choosing organic.

Chapter 10

MEDICAL CONSIDERATIONS REGARDING

WEIGHT

While developing your diet, keep in mind any significant medical conditions which are influenced by how and what you eat. Coronary artery disease, diabetes, Celiac disease, hyperlipidemia, and cancers are some of these diseases. Of course, food allergies also fall into this group.

- Listed below are some of my suggestions:
- Coronary Artery Disease— exclude animal products
- Diabetes— choose foods with the lowest Glycemic Index (G.I.)
- Celiac— avoid foods containing gluten (wheat, rye, barley)
- Hyperlipidemia— foods with low G.I.
- Cancer— eliminate meat and milk products
- Allergies— avoid those foods
- Intolerance— avoid any foods which result in undesirable effects

Surgical Procedures and Weight Loss

Presently, there are three surgical procedures for weight loss. They include banding of the stomach, a partial stomach resection known as the Sleeve procedure, and gastric bypass. All are effective in most patients at least initially, and are suggested for very obese patients with medical conditions benefited by weight loss, such as hypertension, diabetes, and hyperlipidemia.

However, in order to maintain the post-operative weight loss patients must still adhere to some reasonable dietary plan. I prescribe The Dr. Scotti Diet for all of my patients going for these bariatric procedures, both before and after the operations. Those who adhere to the diet almost always maintain the new lower weights.

Medication and Weight Loss

The Dr. Scotti Diet relies on your diet to control weight. Many over the counter substances claim to assist weight loss by various mechanisms such as diminishing appetite, increasing metabolism, creating satiety, and blocking food absorption, among others. None are of proven value and all of the proposed mechanisms are questionable at best.

There have been a number of prescription drugs, many of which were originally approved by the FDA for other uses, which also make claims of causing weight loss. A number of these drugs were initially approved and then taken off the market. The prescription drugs still available and approved for weight loss include Belvig, Qsymia, Orlistat, Didrex, Bontril, and Phentermine.

I have treated patients who have taken over the counter (OTC) drugs as well as approved prescription drugs for weight loss. Many of my patients have also tried prescription drugs off-label for weight loss. "Off-label" means drugs approved for conditions other than weight loss but which have been found to result in decreasing weight as a "side effect" in some patients.

Generally, all of the substances both OTC and prescription, have been of little value in controlling weight in my patients. The one exception in my practice has been prescriptions for Wellbutrin (bupropion) in smokers.

Wellbutrin (an antidepressant) helps decrease the desire to smoke in some smokers. Those who have quit smoking realize that doing so can result in increased appetite and significant weight gain. Many patients, especially women, wil! go back to smoking primarily to decrease the weight gained while off cigarettes. However, those who quit smoking while on Wellbutrin usually do not experience this weight gain and have the added benefit of avoiding the unpleasant change in personality that can follow nicotine withdrawal.

Other than the use of Wellbutrin in smokers, my patients have had essentially no sustained success utilizing diet pills. I will not discourage their use initially for the placebo effect, but I do not consider any kind of diet pill part of The Dr. Scotti Diet or any other program for weight control.

Medications That Effect Weight*

Weight Gain	Weight Loss
Prednisone	Wellbutrin
Elavil	Zonegran
Tofranil	Topamax
Zyprexa	Metformin
Paxil	Phentermine
Zoloft	Concerta
Depakote	Vyvanse
Deabete	Adderall
Diabenese	Strattera
Cardura	Focalin
Inderal	Ritalin
Nexium	Metadate
Prevacid	Valium
Lexapro	Buspar
Prozac	Nardil
BP-Calcium blockers, Beta blockers	Parnate
Clozaril	Byetta
Seroquel	Victoza
Risperdal	Bydureon

Insulin   Qnexa
Tamoxifen   Xenical
Phenelzine   Cymbalta
Valproic Acid   Moban
Gabapentin
Carbamazepine
Lithium

* These medications are used for one of the following diagnoses: depression, psychosis, pain, diabetes, blood pressure, gastro-esophageal reflux disease, breast cancer, seizures, bi-polar disorder. Therefore, if you are on any of these medications and feel it may be affecting your weight, you should consult your doctor.

Chapter 11

Can I drink alcohol on The Dr. Scotti Diet?

Eventually, after you have achieved your target weight, you may drink alcohol. In Stage Four you can add anything you choose. As mentioned in chapter seven, the calorie level of various alcohol drinks varies wildly. As long as you weigh yourself daily and take appropriate action, alcohol need not undermine your weight control.

In fact a little alcohol can sometimes suppress your appetite and help decrease your total caloric intake. The anti-anxiety effects of alcohol can also be helpful for those who are stress eaters.

Can I eat chocolate?

Once you reach Stage Four, nothing is forbidden. Dark chocolate is a good antioxidant and therefore quite healthy. I eat a little dark chocolate in the middle of the day for an energy kick and it also decreases my appetite.

How much weight will I lose?

A 10-12 pound weight loss is not uncommon during the first month on The Dr. Scotti Diet if you follow the plan as outlined. Some patients have lost 50 or more pounds over a three month period.

Must I exercise?

No, but exercise is helpful. What is necessary is motion. Sitting or lying down for most of your waking hours makes weight control much more difficult. If you have a sedentary job or life style, find reasons to move such as doing your own cleaning, yard work, and walking instead of driving.

Is The Dr. Scotti Diet complicated?

Not at all. Just begin Stage One as described by eating only the low fat protein rich foods listed and at least five vegetables each day until you reach your target weight. During this phase, eat all you desire. Once you reach your target, continue to Stage Two and add 1 new fruit each day while maintaining your new lower weight. Stage Three adds grains and Stage Four adds anything else. All must be monitored by daily weigh-ins with adjustments of food intake based on any weight changes.

What if I don't like vegetables?

I have discovered many of my patients don't enjoy eating vegetables. I would encourage you to take the opportunity to try all the possible and available ways to make vegetables tasty. The effort will be worth it when you lose weight and become healthier. Some patients have had success with choosing five vegetables they don't hate, putting them in a blender, and then disguising the taste with added fruit. Also, many of my patients have had success with vegetable soup.

What if I stop losing weight before reaching my goal?

Go back to Stage One, because almost everybody loses weight during that stage. Also have your doctor check you for metabolic problems such as diabetes or an underactive thyroid.

How do I get 5 fruits and 5 vegetables into my diet each day?

Use your imagination! Or, ask others for help and try the following: A blender for fruits and vegetables, vegetable and fruit salads, grilled vegetables, and vegetable soup. Check menus from vegetarian restaurants. Ask a chef.

How do I maintain my weight loss?

Daily weigh-ins. Daily movement. Respond to any weight increase with an honest analysis of why and then correct the problem. Make a list of foods that are Weight Gaining for you and strike them off your shopping list.

Is snacking permitted?

There is no such thing as a snack on The Dr. Scotti Diet. You eat all the low fat protein and vegetables you desire. Eat five handfuls of Weight Neutral or Weight Losing fruits per day once you reach your target weight and the same for grains. When and how often you eat is up to you.

Can I eat beef and/or pork?

Yes, but only if you are not concerned about your health. Red meat and whole milk are some of the least healthy foods because of their association with cancer and heart disease.

Can I eat candy?

Not in large amounts if you want to lose weight and maintain the loss. In small amounts, chocolate can decrease your appetite and even be healthy if you eat dark chocolate, which has antioxidant properties. Non-chocolate candy is a major risk to your weight program and health, so don't even buy it or have any around.

Can I eat in restaurants and stay on my diet?

I do. Once you have mastered your diet and have an acceptable and stable weight you can dine out. Most restaurants have enough menu choices to meet most people's needs. However, fast food restaurants are a challenge and should be avoided by those with questionable will power or who find their diet failing.

How often should I weigh myself?

Every morning (after visiting the bathroom) when you first get up and before eating or drinking anything. This is the foundation of The Dr. Scotti Diet and all of your food decisions are based on your weight.

Should I take vitamins?

Yes, multivitamins help avoid nutritional deficiencies that can create cravings and make you overeat. Ask your doctor to check your blood for deficiencies in iron, vitamin D and vitamin B12, especially if you have cravings. Take vitamins with meals.

Will fruit make me gain weight?

Some may, but not all. By adding a single new fruit each day and checking your weight the next day, you will identify any weight gaining fruits for you. Then, simply don't buy or eat those fruits.

Can I use salt?

Yes, unless you are a salt sensitive hypertensive or have heart failure. Salt plays no roll in obesity and does not have to be avoided.

Can I drink coffee?

Yes, it has no calories and is okay for weight loss if taken without calorie containing sweeteners. Green tea is even better.

What if I don't have will power?

What you need for your weight loss diet is discipline. If you are poor at self-discipline, get someone who can impose some discipline for you via shopping, meal preparation, menu choices, or even a health coach.

Should I share my diet with my doctor?

By all means. If your doctor is overweight she or he may personally profit from The Dr. Scotti Diet. Additionally, as your physician the doctor can perform tests to identify specific food sensitivities, discuss reasons for any food intolerance, find underlying medical problems affecting your weight, and discuss any medical problems you have which may be associated with special dietary needs.

Consult with your doctor prior to any weight loss programs. I recommend you ask for a thorough physical examination, with blood testing. Blood tests should include glucose levels, thyroid function tests, lipids, renal function studies, a complete blood count, iron levels, vitamin B12, and vitamin D levels.

APPENDIX A: QUICK START GUIDE TO THE

DR. SCOTTI DIET

Stage One: Initial Weight Loss

This is the weight-losing phase of The Dr Scotti Diet. Eat **only** low fat proteins (examples listed below) and vegetables. Non-calorie herbs, lemon juice, and condiments such as mustard and vinegar are also permitted. <u>Nothing else!</u> Any and all vegetables are permitted, with the one exception being white potatoes.

Eat as much as you like, do not allow yourself to be hungry, and weigh yourself each morning upon rising. When you have reached your Target Weight goal, you may proceed to Stage Two.

Almost everyone loses weight in this stage of the diet. If, after adhering to this low fat protein and vegetable diet for one or more weeks, you have not lost weight, consult a physician to determine whether or not there is a medical reason for your failure to lose weight.

Example of low fat proteins:
White meat chicken and turkey
Fish - e.g. cod, tuna
Soy products (tofu)
Skim milk
Skim milk products (cheese, yogurt, cottage cheese, mozzarella)
Eggs
Beans

Stage Two: Finding Friendly Fruits
In addition to the low fat protein and vegetable diet you will now begin adding fruits. Add one handful of new fruit daily. Weigh yourself each morning after waking. If your weight has increased <u>at all</u> the morning after adding a new fruit, that fruit is eliminated from your diet. If there has been no weight gain or some weight loss, the fruit can remain in your diet.

Your goal is to find and eat five fruits daily that do not result in weight gain. When you have reached this goal you may move on to Stage Three. If you cannot find five acceptable fruits, eat less fruit and add vegetables until you reach a total of ten fruits and vegetables.

Stage Three: Adding Grains
Foods made from wheat and other gains are a major source of calories and weight gain for most people. This stage is one where you must stick to the principles of daily weigh-ins, adding

a measured amount (one handful) of any single new food each day and eliminating those that result in <u>any</u> increase in weight.

Examples of Grains
Breads
Pasta
Rice
Cake
Cookies
Cereals
Alcohol (substitute 1 drink for a handful)

Stage Four: Adding Everything Else
Adding fats and complex foods not yet introduced to your diet is the final step in the creation of your personalized diet, one that is unique to you. This stage is crucial in the development of a lifelong plan of weight control while enjoying the food you eat. There is no forbidden food, as long as you counter any weight gain with an appropriate Balancing Activity. But you must include the low fat protein and vegetables from Stage One and the fruits from Stage Two in order to have a healthy diet and to prevent overeating of the grains and other foods added during Stages Three and Four.

Remember, the following principals *always* apply:

1. Daily weight recorded each morning
2. Adding a single handful of new food each day

3. Eliminating those causing weight gains <u>or</u> doing some Balancing Activity for foods you love too much to eliminate

APPENDIX B: SUMMARY OF THE

DR. SCOTTI DIET

Stage One: Initial Weight Loss
- Pick target weight
- Eat **only** vegetables and lean proteins (except white potatoes)
- Eat an unlimited amount (until you are full)
- Weigh yourself each morning
- When Target Weight is reached, proceed to Stage Two

Stage Two: Finding Friendly Fruits
- Continue to eat vegetables and lean proteins.
- Add one handful of new fruit daily.
- Weigh yourself each morning.
- If your weight has increased at all the morning after adding a new fruit, that fruit is eliminated from your diet.
- If there's no weight gain or some weight loss, that new fruit remains in your diet.
- Your goal is to find and eat five fruits daily that do not result in weight gain.

- When you have reached this goal you may move on to Stage Three.
- If you cannot find five acceptable fruits, eat less fruit and add vegetables until you reach a total of ten fruits and vegetables.

Stage Three: Adding Grains
- Continue to eat vegetables, lean proteins, and Stage Two fruits.
- Add one handful of a new grain, daily.
- Weigh yourself each morning.
- Eliminate those foods that result in <u>any</u> increase in weight.
- If there's no weight gain or some weight loss, that new grain remains in your diet.
- Move to Stage Four when you've found an acceptable number of Weight/Neutral grains
- If you've found that all grains are Weight Gaining Foods for you, these must be eliminated from your diet or, if you wish to continue to eat them, you must engage in Balancing Activities to counteract the resultant weight gain.

Stage Four: Adding Everything Else
- Continue to eat all foods from Stages One, Two, and Three.
- Add one handful of food not yet introduced to your diet.
- These will most likely be fats and complex foods.
- Weigh yourself each morning.

- Eliminate foods that result in <u>any</u> increase in weight.

- Follow the same procedures as the other stages until you have identified and categorized all foods as either Weight Gaining, Neutral, or Losing for you.

- You will use Balancing Activities to help maintain your weight loss for the long-term.

19112201R00054

Made in the USA
Middletown, DE
04 April 2015